To Melissa

Merry Christmas 2005

Michele CET 1

dog massage

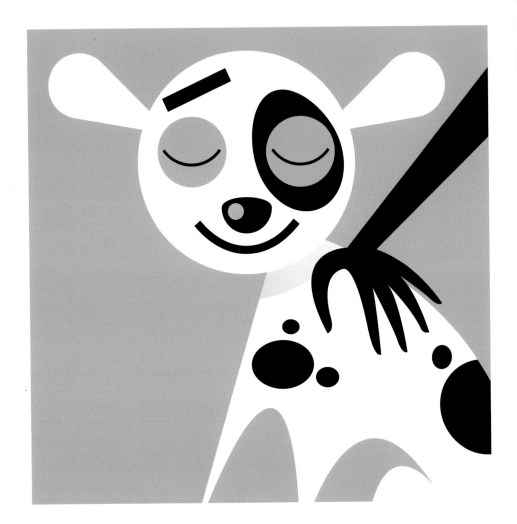

dog massage

expert know-how at your fingertips

Wendy Kavanagh

illlustrations by Bo Lundberg

MQP

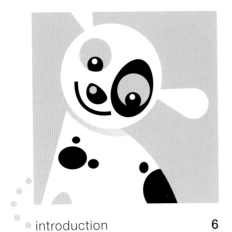

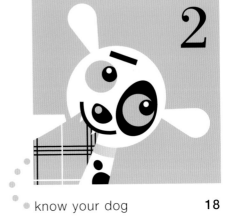

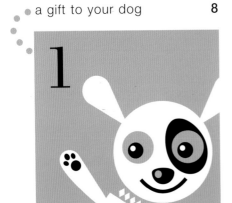

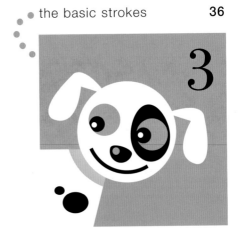

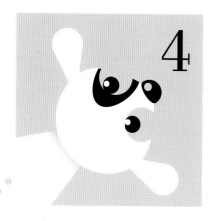

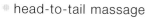

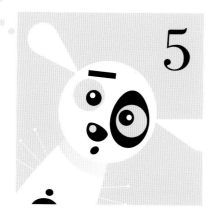

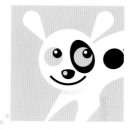

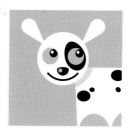

introduction

Whether you're the proud owner of a mischievous mutt or a pedigree champion, learning to use the art of dog massage will make a world of difference to the health and well-being of your favorite four-legged pal. Dogs simply adore being patted and stroked, and frequently nudge you as a reminder to caress and pet them. Now, with this enchanting little book as your guide, you'll be able to direct your touch with expert knowledge.

Massage is the perfect way of caring for your dog, and has many positive benefits—it calms nerves, boosts confidence, improves behavior, soothes aches and pains, stimulates muscle tone, promotes a gleaming, healthy coat, and creates an extra-special bond between you both. What's more, it's good for *your* health too—massaging your dog is a great way of getting relaxed, and can even lower your blood pressure.

Following the detailed, practical know-how, and expert techniques on how to massage every part of your dog's body, from ears to paws, from tail to tummy, you'll soon have your beloved pooch glowing with health and happiness. The case histories described in *Dog Massage* show examples of how massage can help in all kinds of situations, from calming nerves to soothing kennel cough.

The funny, affectionate, and oh-so-knowing illustrations by Swedish artist Bo Lundberg help to guide you through each stage, and capture every nuance of doggy reactions. They are utterly endearing, and will steal your heart as well!

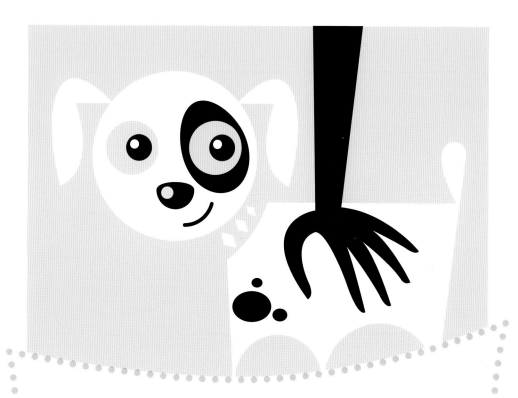

A little note to the reader *In order to avoid constant repetition of the phrase "he or she" in the text, we have referred to the dog as "he" throughout* Dog Massage. *So, if you own a female pooch, be assured that this is entirely arbitrary, and that your pet will benefit from being massaged in equal measure.*

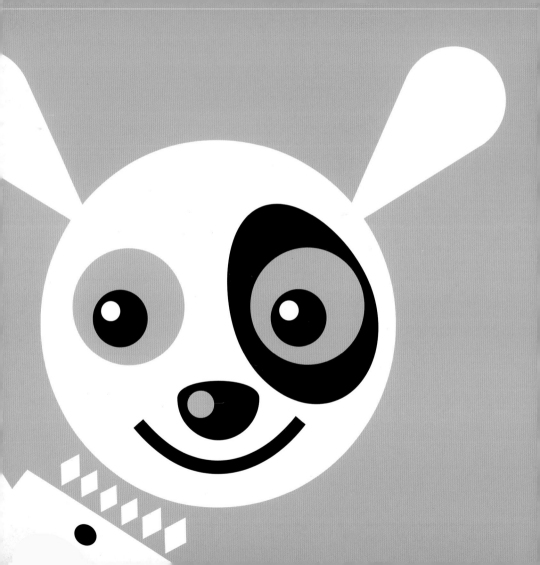

1 a gift to your dog

sheer bliss!

If you've ever had a thoroughly satisfying, relaxing massage, you already know how great it makes you feel. But you may not have thought about the possibility of massaging your dog. Because massage is one of the greatest gifts you can give your faithful pet, it should be an essential part of his routine care.

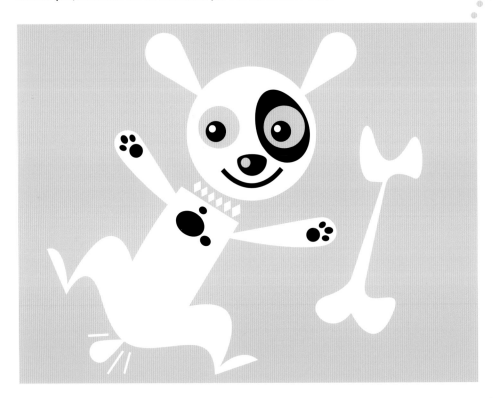

Your dog probably already loves being stroked and cuddled. Massage is effectively a means of formalizing this random petting—with the rewarding result that you will be able to see and feel real, positive changes in your dog's health. It's a great form of preventive healthcare and is a healing and communicative tool literally at your fingertips. Best of all, it's free. All you have to do is give some of your time to learning these loving skills and, as a result, you and your dog will both reap the benefits. Just keep reminding yourself how good massage feels.

Happiness is a relaxing massage from a dog's best friend—and yes, that means you!

This is not just a subjective feeling. During the 1950s, a research project at the University of Wisconsin demonstrated that the experience of being touched was vital for animal well-being. It showed that young animals who were taken away from the litter at birth developed physical, behavioral, and medical problems despite being well-nourished. Both animals and humans need regular physical contact to thrive and feel completely happy.

a timeless art

Massage is a highly focused way of touching; and over the centuries it has gone in and out of fashion as an integral part of health care. As for its role in canine health, historically, it was used almost exclusively on racing and hunting dogs. We know this because a 15th-century illustration shows men caring for hunting dogs with massage. Also, there are beautiful Egyptian wall carvings depicting animal massage. Today, with the recent upsurge of complementary therapies, massage is widely regarded as being as important as good nutrition and exercise in any dog's healthy lifestyle.

mutual benefits

The benefits of massage are essentially the same for dogs as humans. It is a great way to give affection and attention, particularly if your pet spends long periods alone when you are out. Ideally, you should involve the whole family in the exercise. Everyone can take part—you are never too young or too old to massage your dog, and it's a highly effective bonding exercise.

calm and confident

Regular massage encourages your dog to enjoy being handled. It is particularly useful if you can identify the massage strokes your dog seems to like because you can then invite your family and friends to massage him with his favorite strokes. In this way, your dog learns to be confident and to relax and enjoy being handled by different people.

This will help to make visits to the vet less of an ordeal for everyone and is an excellent way to calm and reassure a particularly nervous dog. Aside from making him feel secure and approachable, it is also a wonderful help with your dog's behavioral training. Gradually, you and your dog will become a great "massage team."

Massage is also an excellent early warning system—changes in your dog's physical condition can often be felt before they can be seen. So, by using regular massage, you will notice unusual growths, skin and hair conditions, and the presence of ticks or lice. This gives you a chance to discuss anything of concern with your vet at an early stage.

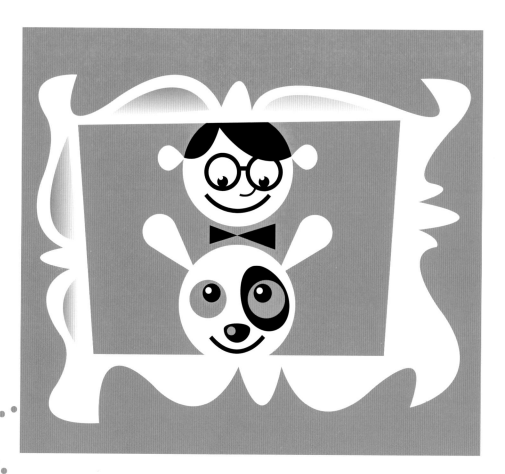

Giving your dog regular massage sessions reduces stress for you both, and creates a loving, trusting bond between you.

13

key improvement areas

In the following ways, massage is a great way of maintaining and improving robust doggy health:

The bones

- Helps with correct posture and balance
- Reduces muscle tension that could lead to more serious problems
- Increases nutrient flow to your dog's bones

Breathing

- Improves breathing patterns
- Helps reduce any respiratory problems

Digestion

- A good remedy for constipation
- Relieves spastic colon
- Reduces water retention
- Cleans the blood by toning the kidneys

Circulation

- Stimulates blood and lymph circulation
- Helps strengthen your dog's immune system
- Releases any toxins held in the body

Muscles

- Relieves muscle tension and spasm
- Removes waste such as lactic acid that builds up after rigorous exercise
- Helps to restore any lost muscle tone and increases joint flexibility
- Increases the flow of blood and nutrients to the muscles

Nervous system

- Relaxes and calms your dog
- Helps your dog to sleep, if restlessness is a problem
- Raises endorphin levels, which promotes healing and a happy disposition
- Safely releases any destructive tendencies that may be held back
- Generally balances your dog's energies

Maisie felt miserable

Maisie and her young owner Charlie were a devoted pair, so it was not surprising that she missed him terribly when he left home for college. Dogs suffer from anxiety, depression, and grief, just like people. And that's what happened to Maisie. She began behaving strangely, and started air-biting, vacant staring, and restless pacing. She also showed classic signs of depression: she became more lethargic instead of wanting to play, and her famous appetite for food was radically upset.

The family decided to consult the vet. He explained that there was nothing physically wrong with Maisie; she was simply unhappy. A friend suggested that Maisie would benefit from massage—so they tried it. The change in Maisie was dramatic. She became calmer, stopped the disturbed behavior, and resumed her usual enthusiastic eating patterns. Her massage sessions reduced her anxiety by relaxing her muscles, and promoting the release of the mood-enhancing, "happy" endorphins. Her overall behavior improved also: a brain chemical called serotonin is related to a dog's confidence, and decreased levels of this neurotransmitter can lead to depression. The improved relationship that touch promotes can be essential in reducing emotional problems. A combination of training, counter-conditioning, and relaxation was highly effective, as Maisie's family discovered. They made a point of associating massage with situations that would normally cause poor behavioral problems, so Maisie became more responsive and willing to cooperate.

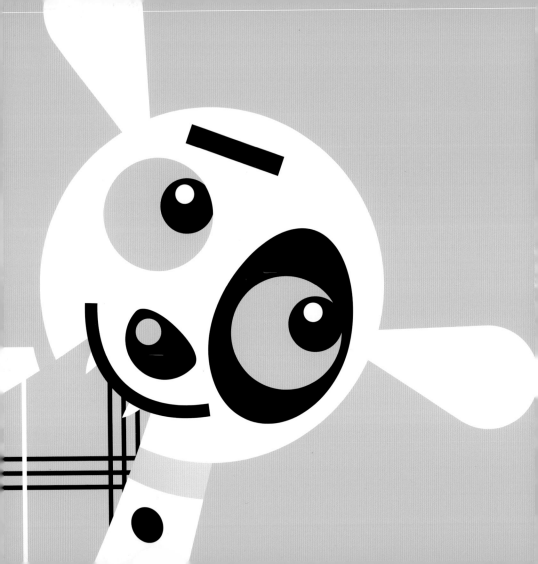

2 know your dog

the working parts

You will develop an instinctive knowledge about your dog the more you massage, but it is always useful to have some basic idea of his body structure and the differences between him and yourself. Think of the areas of your body where you appreciate massage the most—these will be the same for your dog.

The most obvious difference between you and your dog is that you walk on two legs and the dog on four, which positions the limbs quite differently. Aside from this, your major bones correspond, as do the muscles, nervous and circulatory systems, and the functions of the internal organs. If you know where your major muscles and bones are, you can easily figure out where they are on your dog.

Dogs have over 240 bones—approximately 40 more than humans—mostly because of their tails. They also walk on their toes rather than the entire sole of the foot as we do. The primary functions of the bones are supporting the weight of the body, protecting the major organs, and storing essential minerals that the body needs. They also give the freedom of movement to walk, run, or simply curl up and relax. In later years, many dogs experience typical bone disorders such as breaks, slipped discs, and osteoarthritis.

Massage works directly on the muscles, so it helps to know where these are and what they do. Some are situated deep in the body, others near the skin's surface—so you'll need to use different strokes according to which muscle is being treated. Most have Latin names (you may overhear these when visiting the vet). The ones that are directly affected when you massage are listed on the following pages.

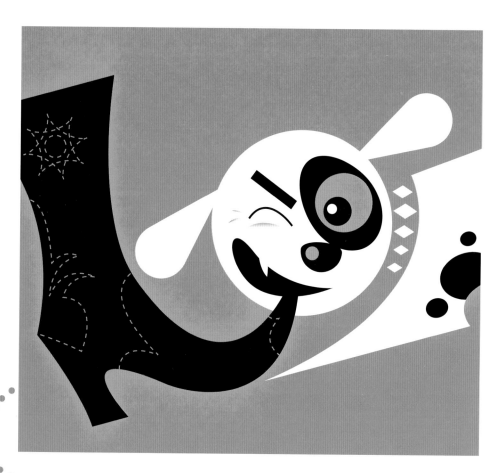

Chewing and biting are a dog's favorite ways of using his head and face muscles—but that can be very hard on your shoes!

canine muscles

Head and face muscles
Functions—chewing, biting, licking, swallowing, facial expressions
Masseter, Buccinator, Temporal

Neck muscles
Functions—turning, rotating, craning
Trapezius, Latissimus dorsi, Brachiocephalicus

Ear muscles
Functions—moves the ears back and up
Auricular

Shoulder and foreleg muscles
Functions—walking, running, stretching, scratching
Biceps, Deltoid, Latissimus dorsi, Trapezius, Triceps

Back muscles
Functions—turning, stretching, raising
Latissimus dorsi, Trapezius

Upper hind leg and rump muscles
Functions—walking, running, jumping, scratching
Biceps femoris, Gastrocnemius, Gluteals

Abdominal muscles

Functions—support the organs of the abdomen

External obliques, Rectus abdominus

Chest muscles

Functions—connect the ribs, flex the shoulder

Intercostals, Pectorals

Forepaw muscles

Functions—scratching, washing, digging

Flexors, Extensors

Tail muscles

Functions—wagging

Controlled by the muscles of the lower back

When you are massaging, you will work on groups of these muscles, using a variety of strokes and focusing on specific points for special therapeutic use.

reading doggy signals

Seeing and hearing your dog's responses will let you know if you are massaging effectively. Watch for the signals that will alert you to what's going on.

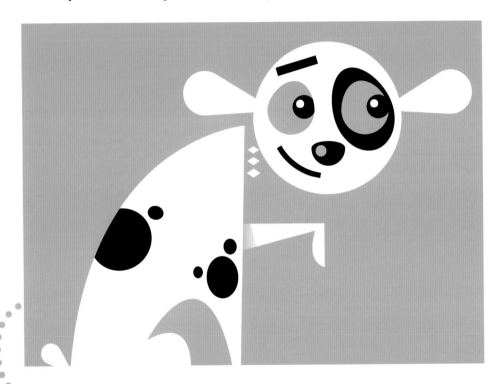

Your dog's body language is loud and clear—he would like a nice massage—preferably now, if you've got a minute.

do and don't

Follow these simple guidelines to ensure that you both enjoy the experience. Think of what you would particularly like or dislike about a massage treatment—the same will probably apply to your dog. Act responsively, listen to your dog, and if you're in any doubt, seek advice from a qualified massage therapist.

Yes, I love it!

Your dog can use a whole range of body language to say that he loves being massaged. His tail will wag; he may lick your hand gently or drift off and drool because he has forgotten to swallow! His face may have a rapt, hypnotized expression, and his loud sighs of pleasure will tell you that you have hit the spot. After you've been massaging him on a regular basis, he may come and ask for a treat by placing his paw on your hand or by rolling over and stretching out invitingly.

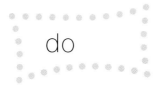

do

- Always have clean, warm hands. Although most dog massage therapists would not advise you to use any oils or creams, there is no harm in occasionally using a very small amount of pure, cold-pressed oil such as a light almond, jojoba, or sunflower. Use it very sparingly to improve your dog's coat if appropriate.

- Make sure that your nails are not too long and do not have jagged, rough edges that will make your dog feel uncomfortable.

- You should always use your hands to massage your dog. Don't try using your feet, for example—you may injure your pet.

- If you have a young dog, massage him after play sessions; otherwise he may become distracted and restless during the routine.

- Always approach gently—sudden movements may make your dog nervous and stressed.

- Stroke and reassure your dog, using the touch he responds to the most. This will calm him down and you will gain his trust in preparation for the massage.

- During the massage, focus your attention on the rhythm of the strokes and your dog's breathing patterns. If you are touching a tender spot or problem area, a sudden change in your dog's breathing may tell you that there's a problem.

- Be aware of the possibility of discovering underlying problems that you may uncover during a massage.

- Listen and feel, taking note of any specific areas that may be uncomfortable to your touch.

- Respect the boundaries your dog establishes and adapt the speed and pressure of your strokes to his current mood.

- Always end the massage promptly when your dog indicates that he has had enough.

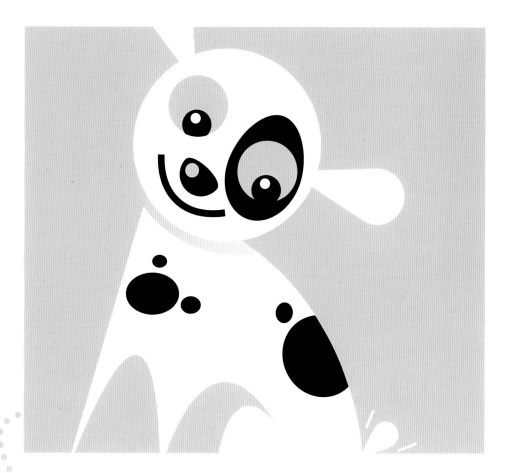

A wagging tail and happy expression leave you in no doubt that your pooch is in a relaxed, welcoming mood.

27

No, I'm not happy!

If he is not happy to be massaged, your dog may growl, bare his teeth, or hold himself rigid. If his ears are flattened back or he pulls away, stop massaging. Any out-of-character behavior might indicate there is an underlying medical problem, especially if he is rejecting strokes he has previously enjoyed. Always pay attention.

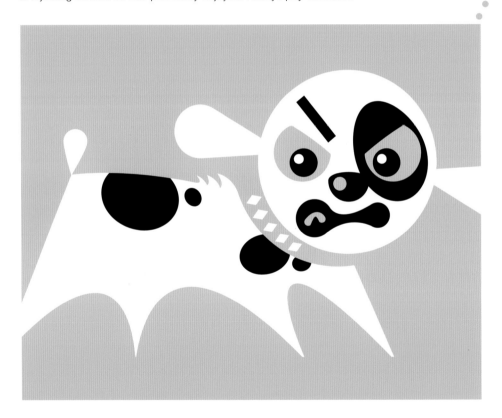

don'ts

When you see this expression on your dog's face, stop immediately. He is telling you in no uncertain terms that he is not happy to be massaged.

- Never try massaging an unfamiliar dog. Both of you need to have an element of trust for this bonding exercise.

- It is not a good idea to start a massage if you are not in the mood or feel unhappy or angry. Your dog will pick up these feelings and will sense that you are not interested in what you are doing. That may make him less responsive to future massages.

- Also, if your dog is not responsive to a massage, don't force him; leave it until he "requests" a treatment.

- During the massage, don't push the limits—listen and sense whether your dog seems happy at all times. Your massage will become very intuitive after a while.

- Don't try to massage your dog if you have used alcohol, sedatives, or non-prescription drugs, because your perceptions will be altered; this is not safe for your dog.

- Start cautiously—don't try giving a full sequence at once. Take plenty of time to allow you and your dog to get well acquainted with this new experience.

- Follow your dog's responses. Don't press so deeply that it is an unpleasant sensation and don't use sudden or jerky movements. Keep your strokes flowing.

- Some places, such as the genital area, are highly stimulating to a dog, so massaging in these spots may over-excite him and make it difficult to conduct a calm massage session. The stomach is also very sensitive—do not press hard on this area.

Do not massage a dog with any of the following conditions:

- Fever, shock, weakness, or exhaustion
- Skin inflammation or infection
- Enlarged glands or swellings of any kind
- Recent skin abrasions or fresh scar tissue

Take extra care in the following circumstances:

- Always work *above* problem areas so that you are not pushing excess blood and lymph into an already aggravated spot.

- Work carefully around the area of recent fractures, sprains, or damaged muscles.

- If your dog has had surgery, wait until he has completely healed before doing any massage.

- Never pull on your dog's fur, ears, tail, or whiskers because this is intensely irritating to a dog.

- Finally, do not use massage as a substitute for consulting a vet. It is a therapy complementary to orthodox treatment—it can enhance, but cannot replace veterinary care.

the right time and place

Never hurry a massage. Instead, make it a calm, measured ritual for you and your dog, and give it an allocated time and place. You might even want to have a special massage mat or blanket to indicate to your dog that it is massage time, much in the same way that he knows it's time for a walk when you reach for his leash. Another way of making it a unique occasion is to reserve a quiet, comfortable place for your massage sessions.

Choose a time that suits you both. It could be at night or at a quiet time in the morning, as long as you and your dog are in the right mood to give and receive. Start off with weekly massage sessions and gradually make it a part of the daily routine.

Think how much better a massage feels in gentle, pleasing surroundings. Soft lighting, relaxing music, and a time away from telephones or televisions all enhance the treatment. Your dog will appreciate the same atmosphere and be more receptive to your touch.

Develop a massage voice, and talk to your dog in quiet, reassuring tones. Praise him for relaxing and develop a key word or phrase to indicate that you are going to start the massage, just as you might say, "Let's go for a walk." If you cannot think of your own phrase, try saying, "touchy-feely time." This soothing, rhythmic, talk will set the tone for the massage and let you check if your dog is receptive before you start.

To prepare yourself, make sure you are comfortably clothed and in a position where you are happy. You could sit on the floor together, or in the case of small dogs, on a chair with your pet on your lap. There is no "official" position; choose one that feels right—your dog will be fine.

Make sure you remove all jewelry, check your fingernails, and relax yourself. Drop your shoulders and shake out your hands. You might want to keep your dog's grooming brush close by to use as a massage tool.

If you have never massaged your dog before and feel a little nervous, you could practice on a pillow or cushion beforehand. The best advice of all is to persevere and if your dog is not initially responsive, try again another time.

You'll find that once your dog becomes familiar with the ritual, he will initiate it by bringing you his massage mat or blanket or by rubbing his head against your hands and looking at you with those "massage" eyes

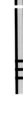

He's brought you his special blanket, and now he's trying to get your attention. How can you resist this appealing invitation to give him a top-to-tail massage? He's using all his charm to get it!

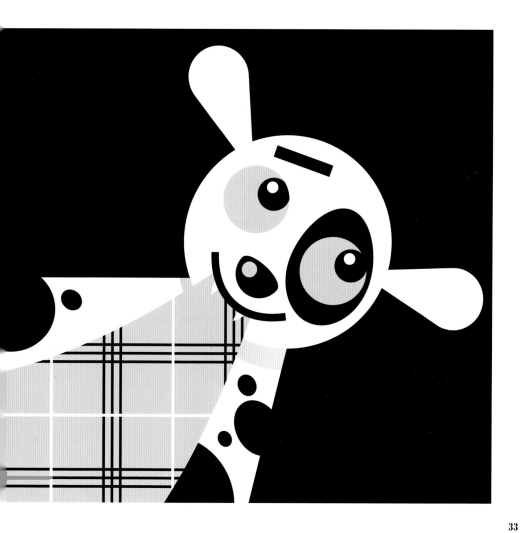

Petra's cough

When her owner was suddenly hospitalized, Petra found herself in kennels for a short while. That's when she picked up kennel cough, the most common problem of the respiratory tract that dogs get. Young dogs are very susceptible to this, because their immune system is immature, but older dogs are also vulnerable. After Petra returned home, she suffered from bouts of high-pitched coughing that kept her and everyone else in the family awake at night for up to 2 weeks. Her nose was obviously blocked up, and she was noticeably in great discomfort.

case history
2

Although there is no cure for kennel cough except time, Petra's owner decided to try massage, after reading that it helps boost and strengthen the immune system and encourages the body to fight disease naturally. Some breeds, such as the King Charles Spaniel, Pugs, and Pekinese, have very small nostrils or elongated soft palates that interfere with respiration. That's why Petra was particularly uncomfortable. To bring relief from her congestion or coughing, her owner massaged her neck and chest areas and over the lungs, lightly tapping with the tips of her fingers to help loosen up excess mucus.

Working on the chest muscles improved Petra's breathing by improving her lung capacity. Her owner boosted the therapeutic effects of the massage sessions by putting an essential oil in a vaporizer in the same room in which she was working. She chose rosemary, but you could also try eucalyptus, which is excellent for helping to clear congestion and soothe a cough.

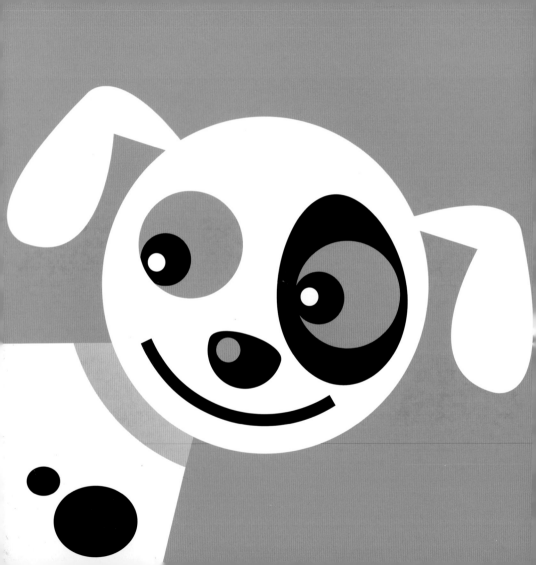

3 the basic strokes

hands-on experience

Make sure that your massage strokes are not too light or tickly. If you have had a massage yourself, you will be aware that there is nothing more annoying than a very superficial treatment. If you have never experienced a massage, it may be useful to have one so that you are aware of what your dog will be feeling.

There are many massage strokes used by professionals, but the basic Swedish techniques are the easiest to learn. It's likely that you've instinctively used some of them when petting your dog.

the holding stroke

Place your hand palm-down in a reassuring manner without actually moving it. Use this stroke at the beginning of the massage to gain trust and indicate what you are about to do. Do it again at the end, to send a signal to your dog that the massage is complete. During the massage, always try to keep one hand in contact with your dog to maintain the flow of trust between you.

palming method

Known professionally as *effleurage*—the French word for stroking—this stroke is done with the hand flat, fingers together, in a gliding movement. Imagine you are swimming the breaststroke, exerting pressure on the upward stroke and reducing pressure on the return.

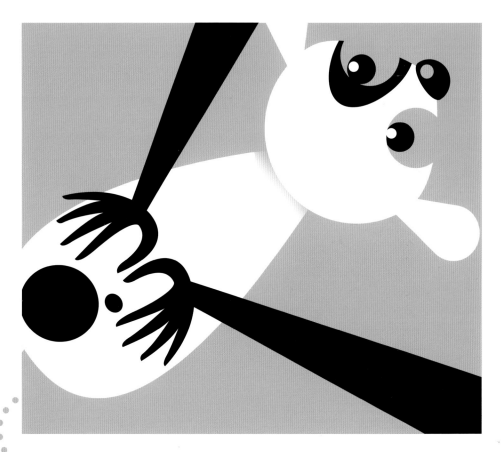

*The palming stroke shown here is so easy to learn, and is
the one you will use most. With practice, you'll soon get it
right—and your dog will love the smooth, gliding, motion.*

Don't break the flow by lifting your hand off your dog's body between strokes. Work along the line of the coat, using one or both hands. For areas such as the tail and thigh, it may be easier to cup your hand against the curve of your dog. This stroke is often used to warm up an area before applying deeper strokes and is great for general relaxation and to massage large areas. Make sure you keep your own shoulders relaxed.

thumb circling and rolling

The pads of your thumbs are used to make very small circles while applying pressure to specific points; you may hardly notice your thumb moving. The circles can be extended as you lean your weight gently into the stroke. You will find that you are able to feel the tissues and muscles under the dog's coat and focus on any "knotty" areas. These are key spots on which you should focus your massage.

When you're massaging your dog, you may often feel patches of tensed, bunched up muscles just beneath the skin. You can release these knotted-up areas by rolling and circling with your thumb, as shown here.

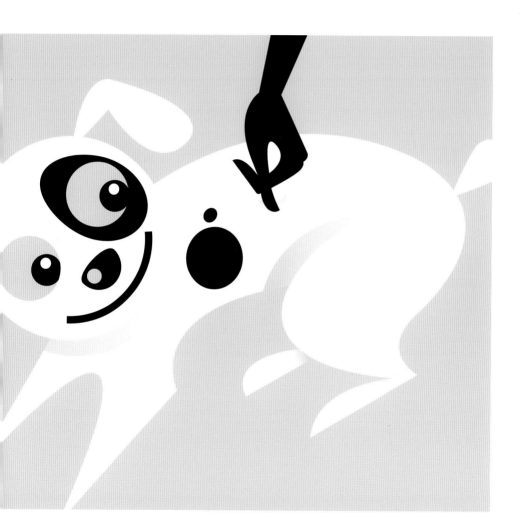

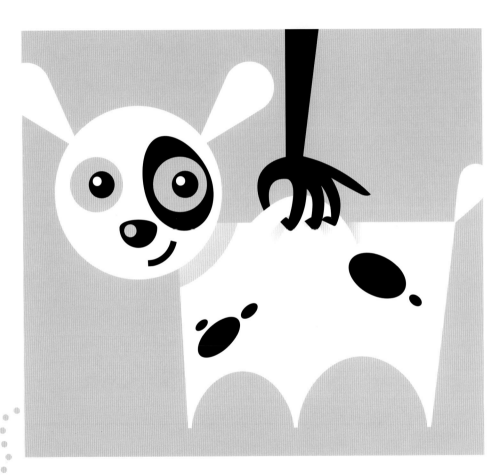

*Your dog's in heaven when you get right under his skin
with this deeply relaxing scoop-and-squeeze stroke.*

To cover larger areas of tension, use the flat length of your thumb to stroke outward, then circle back in a rolling motion. Try this with one hand first and then bring in the other hand; use your thumbs alternatively, as though "twiddling" them over the tense muscle.

You can have fun by varying the speed of this stroke, increasing it to invigorate, and decreasing it to soothe.

flicking stroke

Take care with this stroke if you have long nails. Using only the tips of your fingers, flick very lightly, using one or two fingers, barely making contact with your dog. Even though this stroke is very light, you can actually move the muscle with it.

scoop and squeeze

This is a kneading stroke—*petrissage*—where the muscles are squeezed, rolled, and lifted. Make your hand into a "C" shape, gently squeezing your dog's muscle between the flats of your thumb and forefingers. Use one hand for the massage and support the area where you are working with the other.

The kneading movement should be highly rhythmic—work horizontally across the area, literally milking the muscles of any tension. Practice on your own calf or forearm to check out comfort levels. This is a great stroke to choose for working on the deeper, larger muscles that do all the hard work when your dog runs about.

tapping

A light tapping action is a variation of flicking. Once again, use the tips of one or two fingers, and apply little or no pressure in a vibrating motion. This stroke is often used over larger areas such as the back to release tension. You can change it to a light plucking motion, which is more effective for smaller areas such as the head and neck.

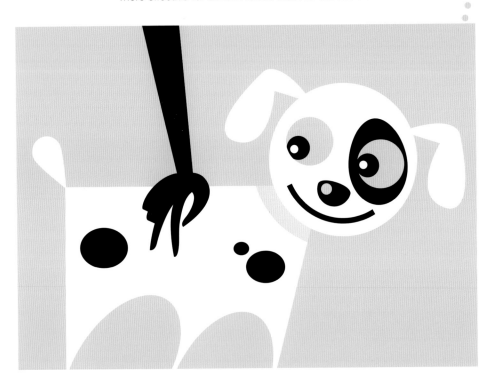

fingers and knuckles

This is a very simple technique and is a natural follow-up to the flat-handed or palming stroke. Use the pads of two or three fingers to apply pressure in a circular movement over the underlying muscle. Maintain contact and widen the circles to cover a larger area as you feel the muscles relax under your hand. Work in a clockwise direction first and then reverse the direction.

If your dog's muscles are all tensed up, use a light tapping action with the tips of your fingers in a steady rhythm.

Working in the same way, now use the undersides of your knuckles to increase the pressure. Bend your massage fingers inward toward the palm of your hand, and make contact with the flat part of the back of the finger, just above the knuckle. Don't dig in with the knuckle ridge itself, because that might be uncomfortable for your dog. You will find that you will be able to move muscles easily with this stroke, and it is useful where more pressure or friction is required.

stroking

This will already be familiar to you because you probably stroke your dog every day. In massage, this light contact uses the undersides of your fingers along broad areas of your dog's body. Always work in the direction of the coat, and, as an enjoyable alternative, fan out your fingers and apply them in a wave-like motion. This is a great way to finish before applying the holding stroke. It calms and settles your dog very effectively—remember how soothing it feels to have loving fingers running through your hair.

Reina and Riva

case history 3

General wear-and-tear and aging often lead to joint problems. Some disorders, such as elbow arthritis in Bernese and Rottweilers, may be inherited. Osteoarthritis is very common in aging dogs, and larger breeds suffer more frequently from it than small dogs. The owner of a fine pair of Old English Sheepdogs called Reina and Riva found that, as they reached old age, both had problems with their hind legs, which made it very difficult for them to get into and out of vehicles or climb stairs. What was done about their problem?

Acupuncture came to their rescue. They both visibly responded to the temporary relief it gave them, which enabled them to spring along like puppies. Massage and "bicycling" their hind legs helped, and trigger point therapy helped to control bone and joint pain. Other breeds, such as Yorkshire Terriers and Golden Retrievers, find that their knee joints suffer more, whereas Toy Poodles are more prone to osteoarthritis in the hip joints. Unlike humans, rheumatoid arthritis is very rare in dogs.

Reina and Riva's owner noticed that Frankie, his friend's Red Setter, was slowing down too. It's not surprising that they hadn't observed this earlier.

Larger dogs are often less sensitive to pain than smaller dogs. They get older but still seem to have the stamina of their youth. As opposed to acute pain, which is sudden and often fleeting, chronic pain is ongoing and associated with aging bones and joints. Sometimes this is hard to recognize immediately because dogs tend to adjust to this type of pain. They can make small changes in their behavior and play patterns, but activities such as climbing stairs will reveal underlying problems. Reina and Riva's owner passed on the tip about gentle massage and acupuncture to Frankie's owner. He tried it and Frankie felt much better.

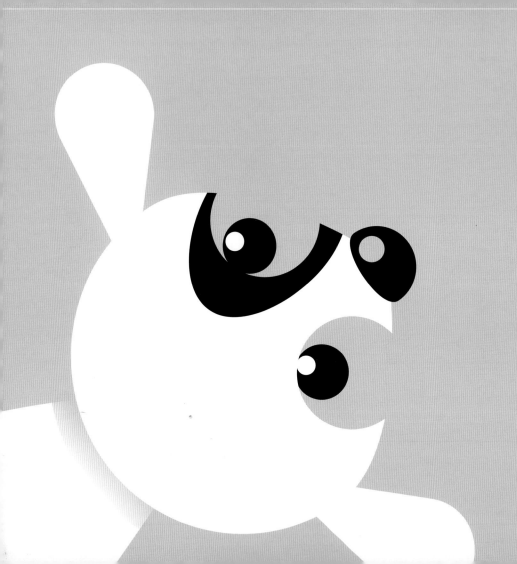

4 head-to-tail massage

head-to-tail massage

Now that you are equipped with the correct techniques, you'll be able to use them in myriad combinations—enough to satisfy your dog's every need. So, go find your favorite pooch and get started. You'll soon discover that magic touch. But don't forget these golden rules: never massage directly over the spine or joints and be careful with sensitive areas like the stomach and kidney region.

Practice makes perfect, so in order to help you and your dog master the art of massage and reap benefits, this head-to-tail massage routine has been split into seven main sequences. They are very easy to learn:

• Top to tail
• Head and face
• Neck and shoulders
• Spine, back and sides
• Chest and belly
• Legs, paws and claws
• Tail

These sessions form a natural sequence, but you can mix and match them once you feel confident. You'll use a variety of strokes because each area has a different bone and muscle arrangement. Your dog will probably like some strokes better than others. You'll get to know which ones they are once massage has become a regular part of your pet-care routine.

By beginning every massage with this well-defined head-to-tail stroke, you'll give your dog a clear signal that this is more than a casual pat.

top to tail

To gain your dog's confidence and to establish contact, start with a simple head-to-tail stroke, remembering to use your special massage voice. With the flat of your hand—the *effleurage* stroke—start at the top of the head and slowly stroke down the length of the back to the tail base. The strokes should be sweeping, with an even pressure, so that your dog can differentiate between this precisely defined massage stroke and a casual affectionate gesture. Repeat these sweeping strokes 4–5 times.

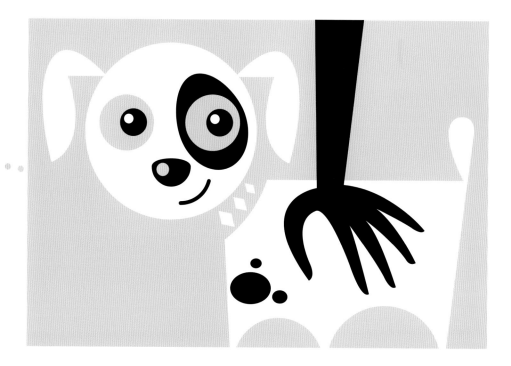

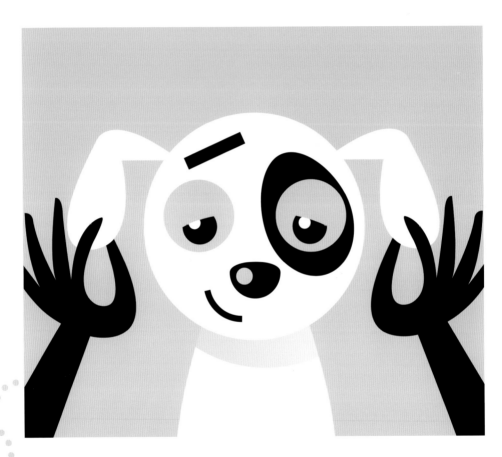

He's so relaxed! Give your dog a treat with this oh-so-gentle ear massage—position your fingers and thumbs exactly as shown, and watch him melt with pleasure.

Repeat these movements, this time including the whole of the tail. When massaging the tail, cup your hands around the base and with a firm but light squeeze, work downward from the base to the tip.

Working within the same area, from your dog's head to the base of the tail, use both hands in an alternate, flowing, and continuous movement. As you lift one hand from the base of the tail, make contact at the head with the other.

Slowly widen the area of this continuous stroke until it becomes a wide glide along one side of your dog, and then the other.

Turn sideways to your dog and place your hands on the shoulder that is farthest from you. Again using the flat-of-the-hand, *effleurage* stroke, alternately stroke outward in a fan-like movement over the shoulder area. You can change the pace and pressure of these strokes if your dog permits. The muscles of the shoulder area work very hard, and massage helps keep them tension-free.

With your dog facing you, place the pads of your forefingers at the back of his neck, behind his ears, and, with light pressure, make small circular movements. Repeat 4–5 times.

Move your hands to the spot under your dog's cheeks and ears and rock his head very gently from side to side. This is a very gentle movement.

If your dog is now relaxed, place your thumb pads about a quarter-inch into the ears with your forefingers on the outer area. Massage his ear gently between your finger pads.

With care, move to the eye area. At this stage, your dog will automatically close his eyes. With the pads of your thumbs, very gently stroke across his eyelids from the inner to the outer edges, working upon both eyes at the same time.

Gently work over the dog's cheeks and mouth, picking up the skin between the pads of the thumbs and forefingers in a very light pinching action. Use both hands alternately if your dog allows it.

Finally, stroke down the dog's throat and chin, using the flat-handed *effleurage* stroke, first with only one hand and then with alternate, continuous strokes.

Once you have mastered this simple head-to-tail routine, you can focus on more specific areas, but remember you should always get your dog's approval before massaging him.

head and face

The head and face are often your dog's favorite place to be touched. He might even invite you to massage him there by stretching his head toward your hand. Because this is such a difficult part of his body to self-groom and clean, your touch is generally very welcome.

You will need to adapt your strokes to the head size of your pet—make them shorter and slower for small dogs, longer and deeper for larger breeds. This will become instinctive the more you massage.

Cautions:

- The windpipe—avoid pressure
- Whiskers—don't bend them forward
- Cheek and teeth area
- Around the ears, particularly with shorthaired dogs
- Any unfriendly responses

Don't forget to use your special "massage" voice throughout the session, so that your dog feels calm and relaxed. To instill a feeling of trust, start working gently and slowly under the chin. Using the pads of your fingers, begin massaging by stroking lightly from the throat to the chin in both directions. Notice the muscles along each side. These are important, as they are used to flex the head and extend to the base of the skull at each ear.

Still using your finger pads, work all over this area in small circular movements, remembering not to put pressure on the dog's windpipe.

Next, with your hand cupped, use your open palm to work from the dog's throat to his chin and across the area. If your dog is comfortable with this, add a gentle squeeze so that you slowly scoop and squeeze upward and stroke downward.

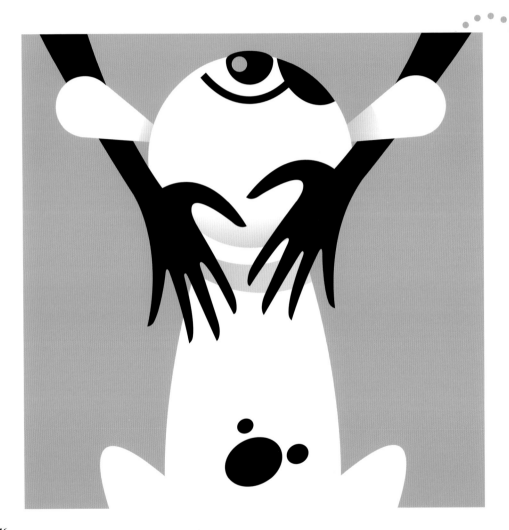

If your dog stretches his head and chin upward while you're massaging him, he's showing his approval. It's a sure sign that you are doing well and that he's very happy.

The next step is to begin the head massage. Use the flats of your fingers and gently stroke backward from the dog's muzzle several times. You probably do this naturally when petting your dog. While you are stroking this area, you'll be working on the temple muscles of his head. These are very powerful and are located on either side of the head in front of each ear, just as in humans.

Using your finger pads and tips, or the flattened knuckles on one hand, and supporting the dog's head with your other hand, massage in small circular movements over this area and the entire top of the head. Work clockwise, varying your pressure.

You can also adapt the speed and size of your circles. Watch closely. You might notice that your dog starts to move his head and even close his eyes in response to your touch.

Next, using gentle flicking strokes, work across the top of the head from the center to the ear base and back. This can be uncomfortable for a dog with a short coat. If he gives you an unfavorable response, move on so you don't disturb the flow of the massage session.

Place your hand on your dog's forehead, your palm on the crown. Then, with flattened fingers, stroke up and down and across the dog's forehead, and end in a circular movement. Work the area from the nose to the top of the head. Your dog will often lead you in this stroke because he knows what he likes.

During the massage sequence, you can pause at intervals by resting your dog's head in your cupped hand, taking all the weight. You can also use the backs of your fingers, with the knuckles slightly bent, to support the chin. This is a favorite position for dogs—they love to rest their heads and relax and would love to choose a nearby lap.

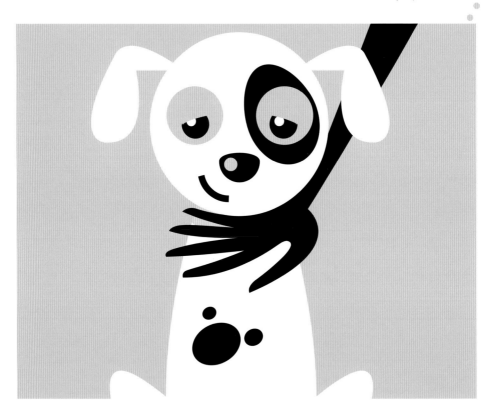

A dog's jaw muscles are often difficult to work with, but it's important to relax them. Cup one hand under his chin and the other over his forehead and use your forefinger to massage one side and your thumb on the other.

Move to the side of the dog's head, under and behind the ears, and use flattened knuckles to make very tiny clockwise circles. Be careful of the ear opening and support his head with your other hand.

To provide a relaxing moment during the massage, let your dog's head rest on the backs of your fingers. He'll really love doing this, as it is a calming, trusting gesture.

Slow down and use your finger pads to stroke over the dog's cheek area, alternating circular movements with short stroking motions. Take special care in this very sensitive spot. The whisker beds are situated in this area, so make sure you do not bend back the whiskers. Instead, smooth over them with the flats of your fingers.

Start from the tip of the nose, using a light but non-ticklish pressure, and work very slowly. Always apply this stroke after you have worked on the head for a few minutes and relaxed your dog. If he shows any signs of discomfort, stop and move on.

Don't forget your dog's cheeks, or *buccae*, as they are professionally known. He'll enjoy this new experience. Facing your dog and using both hands, place the palms of your hands on either side of his head at the base of his ears.

Bring your thumbs inward and place the fleshy part of your hands below your thumbs, on each corresponding dog cheek behind the whiskers. Use this area of your hand to massage back and forth with short strokes, followed by circling motions, first clockwise and then counterclockwise.

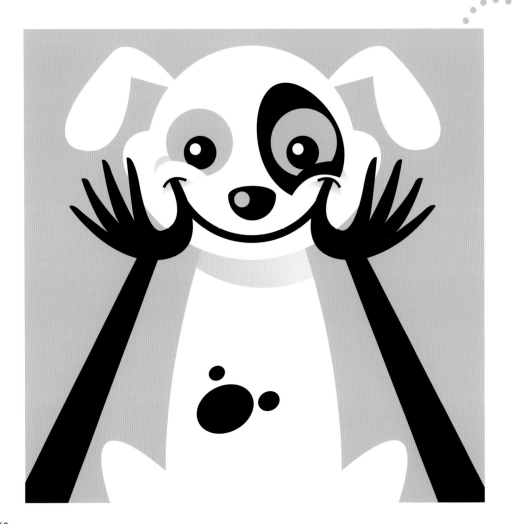

You and your dog will have great fun with a cheek massage. How much more pleasure can this cute pooch take?

When you're more proficient, you can even massage each cheek alternately. This means that when your left hand is at the top of the cheek area, your right hand is working the bottom. Massage slowly and gently so that you do not startle your dog.

Finally, finish by returning to the top of the dog's head and resting your hands on it with a slight pressure before removing them. This will clearly indicate to your dog that the head and face massage is complete.

neck and shoulders

As with humans, massage in this area has a very relaxing effect. Because dogs use their neck and shoulder muscles in most activities—sniffing along the ground, stretching their heads upward to get your attention, observing their surroundings—aches, pains, or muscle fatigue often occur here.

The neck is probably the part of your dog's body that you touch the most every day. However, a little change in the way you use a stroking action can bring the powerful benefits of a massage.

Cautions:

• Never work directly on the spine
• Don't use too much pressure when massaging small dogs
• Don't push the neck or head forward

With the palm of your hand, use a gliding stroke and work from the neck to the shoulders, applying pressure on the downward stroke. Apply five or six strokes on each side and continue using the pads of your fingers, the flats of your knuckles, and the pad of your thumb. For variation, snake your fingers down and along the sides of his neck, changing pressure and speed. Pay attention to what your dog prefers and give him more of the same.

Turn your hand sideways and cup it over the top and sides of his neck. Glide your hand slowly downward, once again with pressure on the downward strokes. Your dog may press his neck into your hand, inviting you to work deeper. His mood will determine whether he prefers a slow or invigorating massage.

In this sideways position, open your cupped hand to form a web — with your thumb on one side of the dog's neck, and your fingers on the other. With the palm of your hand resting over his spine, work down his neck in small strokes by very gently squeezing, pulling up, and releasing the muscle between your thumb and fingers. Be careful not to pinch your dog, though! Just use a very light scoop and squeeze action and watch your dog melt!

Using the flicking stroke, work up and down the neck area on either side of the spine, finishing at the top of the neck. Then, with the pads of your fingers, massage in tiny circles over the base of the skull. Don't forget to support the dog's chin with your other hand. You can also cradle the base of his skull in the web of your hand and slowly draw together your thumb and finger pads, working along the edge of the bone. Finish this stage with a good, long stroke from head to neck before moving on to the shoulder.

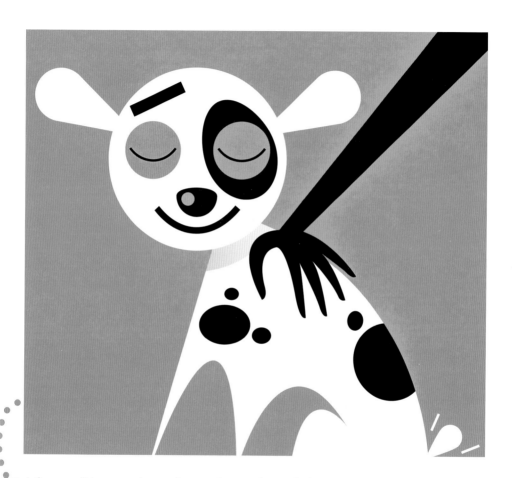

A firm, confident, cupping stroke over the top of your dog's neck is deeply soothing, relaxing, and reassuring.

The shoulder is one of the most important areas to massage. It bears most of a dog's weight, acts as a shock absorber, and is always working when your dog is moving. You can feel the major bone, the scapula, with its prominent edges, on both sides of the body.

With your dog sitting, standing, or lying on his side, glide downward over the area a few times with the palm of your hand. As you do in the neck area, repeat this stroke, using different parts of your hand, including the pads of your fingers, flattened knuckles, and the fleshy base of your thumb.

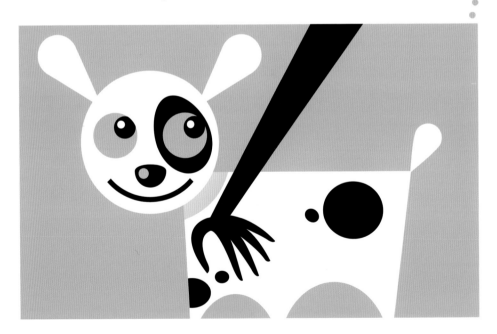

Get to know your dog's shoulder blades. On upward strokes, try a combing action with your finger pads and increase speed in a more playful manner. Use a snaking or circling motion over the whole area. This is a great place to work vigorously and have lots of fun doing it.

Hold your dog's foreleg in a web made from both of your hands and glide downward toward his paw, then move upward again; do this a few times. Next, supporting the leg on your palm and fingers, use the flats of your thumbs in a small rolling motion, one following the other, alternating speed and pressure over the base of the dog's shoulder bone. Don't forget that he has a shoulder bone on each side. Whatever you do on one side, repeat it on the other.

Your dog's shoulders have to do a lot of work, so they often get tense and sore. That's why he will really appreciate a deep, thorough massage session in this area.

Placing both hands flat—on both sides of the dog's spine—massage clockwise in small circles along the shoulders. Gradually make the circles larger until your massage reaches the edges of his shoulder blades. Change direction, working counterclockwise, and then move your hands alternately so that when one hand is at the top of the shoulder, the other is at the base.

Taking the index finger and middle finger of one hand, place the pads on either side of the spine. You will feel a groove between the shoulder blade and the spine that your fingers can naturally follow from the neck to the shoulder. Glide up and down, working very slowly and gently.

Finally, as you work down this groove, feeling the muscles and tendons, press the pads and tips of your fingers at specific points and hold for a few seconds. Then slowly make very tiny circles that are almost motionless and release them. Finally, finish with a few gliding strokes with the palms of your hands over the dog's shoulder area.

spine, back, and sides

To gain your dog's confidence and to establish contact, start with a simple head to tail stroke. Using the palms of your hands, place them on either side of the dog's spine and starting at the top of his head, slowly stroke along the length of his back to the base of his tail. Make sweeping strokes with even pressure so that the dog can differentiate between a massage stroke and a casual, affectionate gesture.

Do not massage directly on your dog's spine. When massaging with your fingers and thumbs, as shown here, position them carefully on either side of the spine, and work on one small area at a time.

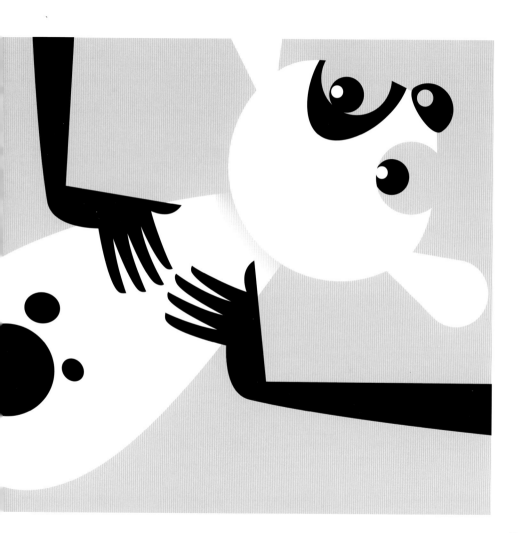

Working in the same area, use two hands in an alternate, continuous movement. As you lift off from the base of the tail with one hand, make contact at the head with the other.

Next, position your finger pads on either side of the dog's spine, to the side of the ridges that you can feel. Then, covering only a small area at a time, rub with your thumb pads. Repeat this action all the way down the spine to the base of the tail, and return.

As you work in this area, you will feel the thick muscles on either side of the spine that are so important to your dog's range of movement. It is very important to keep these muscles relaxed and toned.

Make small circles with your finger pads, over and along these muscles, first clockwise and then counterclockwise, without lifting your fingers. Use more pressure if your dog is happy.

Your dog's size and reaction to this stroke will let you know what is comfortable for him. The more you massage, the more sensitive your touch will become.

As a variation, use a light, rhythmic tapping action along the area with the tips of your fingers—but not if you have long fingernails! This is a good way of releasing muscle tension.

If your dog seems well relaxed and is happy for you to continue, take a roll of skin between each of your thumbs and your first two fingers and lift and knead it at the same time. This stroke can be highly invigorating and enjoyable for a dog.

chest and belly

Start at chest level and work down, incorporating the belly. You can massage the chest area from several positions. Your dog can sit or lie on one side, and then the other, or he can lie on his back with his head and neck cradled in your lap. Your choice depends primarily on your dog's size.

Working from the bottom of the dog's throat area in a horizontal direction, apply finger pads, fingertips, and then flattened knuckles to cover the whole chest region. Vary the pressure and direction in which you are working. Use circling and gliding strokes to work vertically across the dog's chest. Locate the center of his breastplate and rub around the area slowly. This is a gentle, playful sequence.

With your fingers together and your hand slightly cupped, hold his chest in your palm for a moment. With a small dog, you'll be holding the whole chest. For a larger dog, squeeze it with your palm a few times.

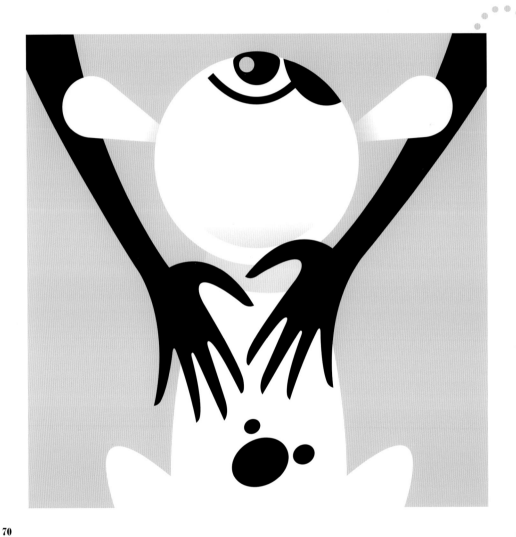

A gentle massage of his chest and breastbone area has a deeply soothing effect on your dog. Watch his face—it will have an expression of pure bliss.

Repeat those movements until you have covered the dog's entire chest. You will feel his pectoral muscles—use the palms of your hands. With your dog lying on his side, keep one hand on his head, shoulder, or hip to calm and reassure him, and use the other hand, with your fingers spread open, to start stroking downward from the shoulder blade and over the chest.

After familiarizing yourself with the area, follow each rib from the spine to the breastbone, massaging the muscle between these bones. Finish with some light strokes, using the palm of your hand to soothe the area following the line of the coat.

While you are working here, don't forget the dog's underarm. Glide your way up to the armpit and, with your other hand, lift his front leg up and slightly away from the chest; this lets you circle, glide, and even very lightly flick over the exposed area. Your dog will show his enjoyment by reaching out for more, so don't forget the other side.

Now that your dog is at ease and receptive to touch, you can start to massage his more delicate belly region. Start with a gliding stroke and, using the palms of both your hands, cover the whole area of his belly including the sides.

Work in a clockwise direction when you are circling because this is the direction of the digestive flow, and is more comfortable for your dog. Use different parts of your hands to do this, alternate the size of your circles, and even include some tickling. Think of the comfort you get from having your own belly rubbed. It has the same effect on your dog. With smaller dogs, you might want to use only one hand. With the palm of your hand, hold his belly in the web between your thumb and fingers.

With smaller dogs, you might want to use only one hand. With the palm of your hand, hold his belly in the web between your thumb and fingers and slowly knead the area with a soft scoop and squeeze motion. Be careful near the pelvic area, where the bladder and kidneys are located.

If your dog wants to end the session, he may simply sit down or stand up. While he is standing, use the palms of both hands to glide gently backward and forward, and from side to side, in a playful manner, finishing with a few short rubs.

There's nothing like a friendly belly rub to put a dog in the happiest mood imaginable. He will literally wriggle and roll about with joy.

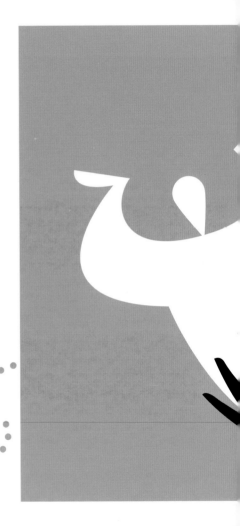

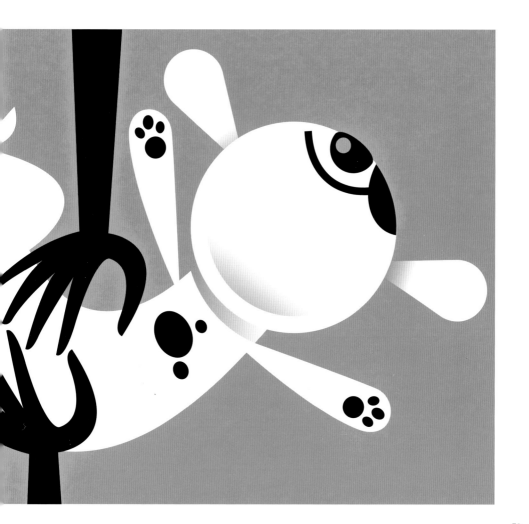

legs, paws, and claws

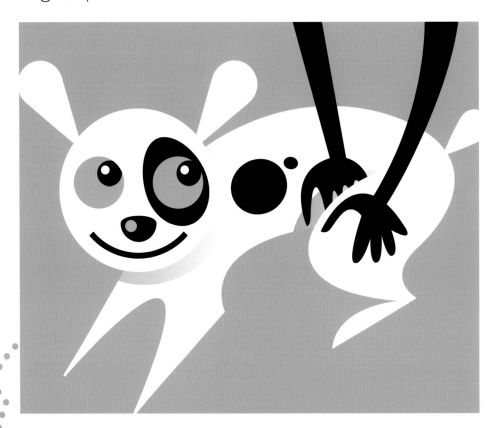

*Mmm, that's wonderful! The expression on your pooch's face
tells you that this hind leg massage really hits the spot.*

Cautions:

• Keep your touch gentle
• If you receive any negative feedback, stop the massage
• Warm up the paw area before touching the claws

Hind leg

The thigh contains several major muscles and can easily take deep massage strokes. These muscles enable your dog to move forward, jump, and leap high in the air.

With your dog in a sitting or lying position, place the palms of your hands on either side of the thigh of his hind leg. With your thumbs pointing down toward his foot and his leg resting on your upturned palm and fingers, slowly stroke across the area, using one thumb and then the other in an alternate rolling action.

Vary your speed and pressure, working the entire thigh area. Change the roll to a circular movement, keeping the circles small and focused. If you flex and extend the leg occasionally, you will be able to locate the hip joint and the inside thigh.

Supporting the dog's foot with one hand, take his leg between your thumb and fingers of your other hand and gently squeeze along the leg muscles. You can use straight or circular movements. Pay attention to the areas around the knee joint and hock, or Achilles' tendon.

Foreleg

Start with a few gliding strokes over the dog's shoulder area and with one hand supporting his foreleg, massage the main muscles. Use your fingers and thumbs, as you did for the hind leg.

When you reach the elbow, flex and extend the leg a couple of times and apply some deep strokes and squeezes around the joint. At the wrist, knead crosswise and, holding the paw, flex and extend his foreleg to help relax and stretch the tendons.

With both the hind and forelegs, massage upward toward the thigh or shoulder with deep pressure. On the downward stroke, moving toward the paws, be more gentle.

Paws, claws

Dogs use their paws and claws as people use their hands and fingers; they are constantly moving and are used for everything from scratching to maintaining traction. A dog's fore paws correspond to our hands and the hind paws to our feet.

You can massage the dog's paws as a continuation of each leg, with him sitting or lying down.

When you have worked his upper leg, continue to squeeze the muscle between the thumb and finger pads of one hand and support the upper leg with the other hand.

Many muscles lie between your dog's toes, so work between each toe by very gently moving up and down a couple of times.

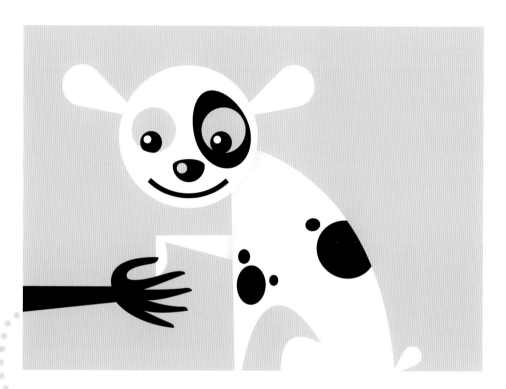

Your dog offers you his paw to show you his trust. Reward him with a gentle and thorough foot massage.

Finish by letting your dog's paw rest in the palm of your hand. Then slowly rotate your fingers clockwise, covering the whole of the pad of the paw. Take it in a classic handshake position and gently squeeze and glide off the paw.

Don't forget your dog has four legs and paws, so remember to massage each of them!

finally, the tail!

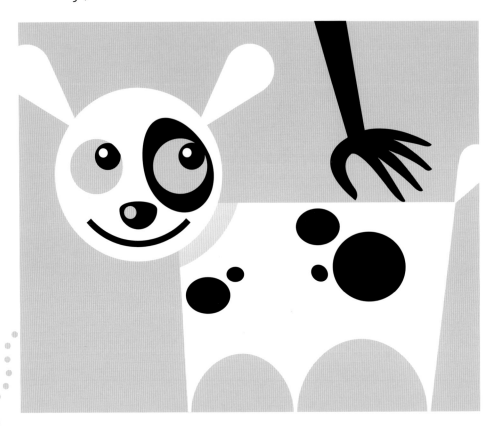

Happy dog, happy tail! That's the gratifying end result of a top-to-tail massage completed to the satisfaction of you both.

Cautions:

- Keep your touch gentle
- If you receive any negative feedback, stop the massage
- If the dog's tail becomes tense or drops between his legs, stop massaging

Start around the base of the dog's tail, formally described as the rump or sacral area. The human sacrum is made up of five bones, but your dog has up to 22 bones—they form the tail.

You will feel a "space" between his pelvis and tail, surrounded by powerful rump muscles. With the pads of your fingers, use very light strokes in a circular motion over these muscles. This area can be hypersensitive, so be careful.

Next, take his tail in the web made of both of your hands. Between your thumbs and fingers, gently feel along the tail to its end. Return and work the length of his tail again, this time gently rubbing between the pads of your thumbs and fingers as you move along.

Finally, stroke gently and steadily down the length of the tail with the palm of one hand, supporting it from the underside with the other hand and gliding lightly off the tip.

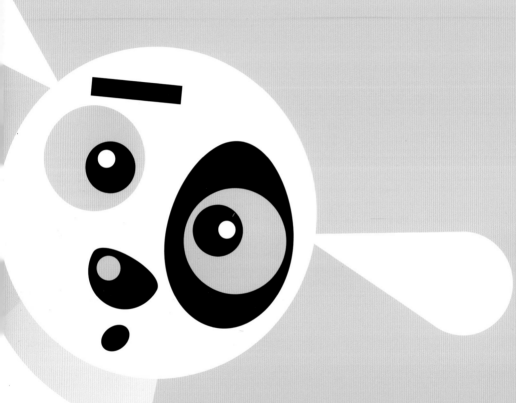

5 special treatments

gently does it

Specialized canine massage therapists can evaluate your dog's needs, if necessary. They begin by asking you to walk and then trot your dog so they can observe his posture and movement. They also ask questions about attitude, past health, and eating habits. Finally, they will recommend suitable therapeutic methods.

Aging dogs Older animals really appreciate the gentle touch and time you give to them during a massage session. Massage releases the "feel good" endorphins that are sometimes referred to as the body's built-in pain relievers. For dogs suffering discomfort from arthritis, hip dysplasia, or joint problems, massage can bring improved comfort and well-being. If a geriatric dog cannot sit for long periods, massage therapy and a set of specialized exercises may improve his ability to hold a sitting position. You can adjust this routine according to the state of health of your dog. Remember, too, that some days will be better than others.

Older and heavy animals benefit from massage around the elbow joints, which often become points of chronic lameness.

Stimulating blood and lymph circulation with massage is beneficial to older dogs with impaired heart function. Five minutes of gentle, flat-handed massage—working upward toward the heart from the dog's extremities—followed by a short invigorating treatment, can help.

Behavioral problems Touch can play a major role in helping dysfunctional or hyperactive dogs, because it reduces anxiety and releases happy, mood-enhancing endorphins. Together with the bonding that occurs between dog and owner, you can include massage in any obedience-training program.

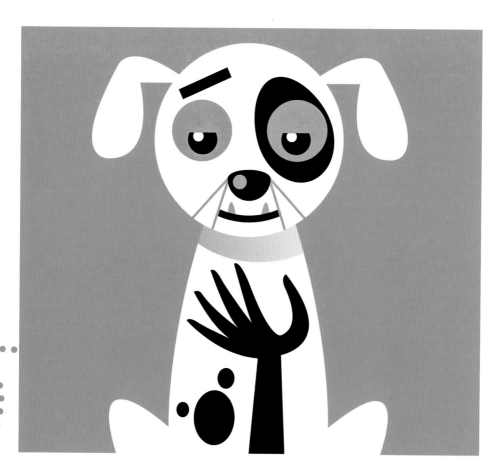

The years may bring many aches and pains to your dear old pooch, so massage is a loving way of bringing blessed relief.

Growing puppies As with human babies, massage is known to help growth, particularly in premature births. Swedish studies of dogs have shown that "massaged" pups grow faster and are healthier than their counterparts.

Large dogs The larger breeds of dog are often prone to minor sprains and strains. A few minutes each day of localized massage in the joint regions will encourage growth and calcification.

Pregnancy The extra weight that dogs carry during pregnancy can bring aches and pains, particularly backaches. Do the massage with your dog lying on her side but use only gentle, flat-handed strokes on her back and stomach areas.

Post-injury and illness Massage can relax and help your dog's own self-repair mechanism to work effectively. In an area where a muscle, tendon, or ligament is injured, you can use massage to stimulate the blood flow to the muscles and organs. This also helps eliminate toxins, such as lactic acid, that build up. After an illness, massage helps the dog's body to recover by stimulating the various physiological systems that keep a dog healthy.

Racing and show-dogs You can make noticeable changes by combining massage techniques such as *effleurage* and cross-fiber friction. Use a general massage before you focus on any problem areas. Sports massage will increase circulation and bring fresh blood to the muscles. As it does with people, it may also increase a dog's performance. It's very common to massage show-dogs, because it can have a positive effect on obedience and conformation

He's a winner because he is in tip-top form. A massage session helps him to relax on the big day, so that he feels calm and confident.

Pre-event massage This is a short, non-invasive session. Use a very light technique to warm up your dog's muscles before a class or race. This massage can also relax or stimulate him and prepare the soft tissues for the event.

Post-event massage This massage technique helps cool down the dog and lower his breathing rate. It can also help reduce the build-up of toxins that can give some muscle discomfort after a race. This is particularly important because muscular discomfort can make your dog resistant or unwilling to move.

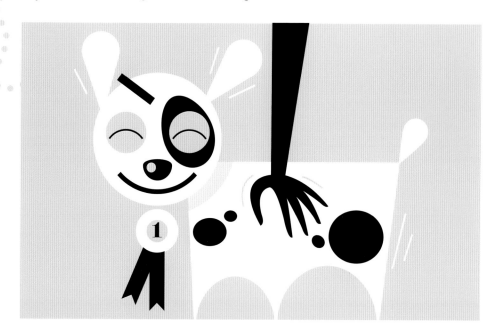

other touch therapies

Acupuncture

A traditional Chinese treatment, veterinary acupuncture dates back over 3,000 years and has been documented in an ancient treatise on the use of acupuncture on elephants.

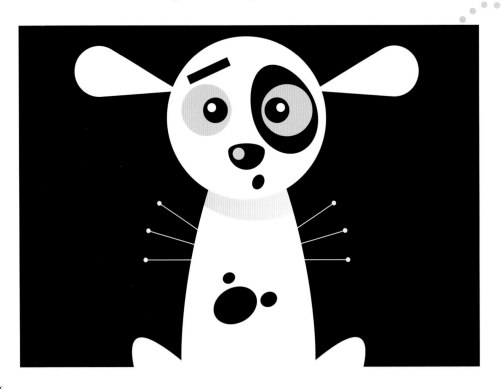

Acupuncture is based on a theory that the body has a life force, or *qi*, that flows along meridian or energy lines. The *qi* keeps the body in perfect balance and health. Acupuncturists insert very fine needles at points along the meridians to stimulate or suppress energy. Although humans have 670 of these points, dogs have only 112.

Acupuncture is most frequently used for pain-related problems, such as arthritis, tendon injuries, and back pain. Some veterinary acupuncturists use the method to enhance healing, and they say that, on the whole, dogs accept needle insertion.

Sticking pins in your pooch? Well, no! These are very fine acupuncture needles. The treatment won't hurt your dog—on the contrary, it is excellent for relieving arthritis and muscle pain.

Acupressure

Acupressure works just as acupuncture does and possibly predates it. Instead of needles, you use your fingers to apply a steady pressure (tuina) to the acupressure points. The Japanese developed a similar form of massage, known as *anma*. Vets use this technique on dogs that have an aversion to needles. They may also use it to relax a dog before working with acupuncture. Dog owners can also use it to maintain therapy between visits to the specialist.

Chiropractic

Chiropractic practices were developed in Canada in 1895 by Daniel Palmer. In the 1950s, a British chiropractor, John McTimoney, adapted a more gentle form of this treatment to use with animals. Chiropractic practitioners believe that the backbone is the key to making the entire system of muscles, joints, and bones function smoothly. Chiropractors examine the spinal column and pelvis and use their hands to manipulate and palpate appropriately. Although few vets use chiropractic care for animals, some specialists use it successfully to treat dogs, such as greyhounds. Short-legged or long-backed breeds may also benefit from chiropractic therapy.

Hydrotherapy

Vets in Hakone, Japan, were the first to use hydrotherapy for treating dogs. Since then, the practice has spread worldwide and specialist canine spas have been established. Water is an ideal medium for hot and cold treatments and is often used to stimulate muscles and joints after injury or surgery. Cold water redirects blood to the internal organs to help them function better, whereas hot water increases blood flow to the muscles and skin, helping circulation and easing stiffness. Where facilities are available, vets often refer injured dogs to hydrotherapists. They may also suggest it as a form of physiotherapy.

Just lie back and enjoy it! The pain-relieving benefits of hydrotherapy are widely recommended for treating muscular injuries.

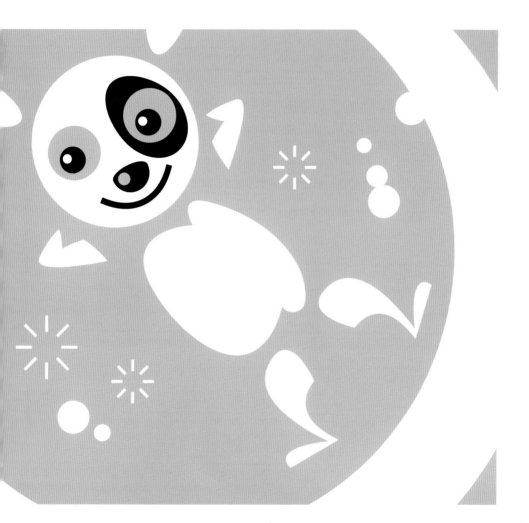

Osteopathy

Developed by Dr. Andrew Taylor Still, who founded the American School of Osteopathy in 1892, osteopathy uses touch to treat all parts of the body's structure. Unlike chiropractic, which only deals with the spine, osteopathy's aim is to work on soft tissue by using manual manipulation to relax the muscles and thereby increase mobility.

Nowadays, increasing numbers of practitioners who specialize in working with dogs are exploring methods similar to those traditionally used for humans. Osteopaths have had good results in many cases, particularly with dachshunds, as they tend to suffer from back pain; but little documented research has been conducted.

TTouch therapy

In 1978, a Canadian horse trainer named Linda Tellington-Jones adapted an older touch therapy, the Feldenkrais Method, to use on her horses. She later applied the technique to dogs, cats, and other animals. In 1984, she introduced TTouch, a gentle therapy that works only at skin level. Using relaxed fingers, you make circular motions, and tailor your motions to each particular dog. The method is widely used to calm nervous dogs and helps with training by relaxing and focusing animals. Used widely in the US, Canada, and the UK, either a TTouch therapist, vet, or dog owner can use it.

Trigger point therapy

Originating in China, but adapted by Western conventional medical teaching, this technique treats muscle pain. Pain is not always felt at the site of an injury; frequently it is experienced at a referred point.

In this technique you apply firm pressure to these points, which may result in initial discomfort, but is followed by release and pain relief.

Because muscle tissue tends to be neglected by other therapies, it is prone to damage. A dog's weight is made up of over 40% muscle. You may have noticed your pooch instinctively moving his weight to avoid using a painful leg. The response to Trigger Point Therapy is fast for recent problems and a little longer for chronic pain.

Shiatsu

Based on the same principles as acupuncture and acupressure, this technique was introduced to Japan over 1,500 years ago. Dog shiatsu is practiced widely there today, as it is in Australia. Literally meaning "finger pressure," the treatment covers the entire body, stimulating muscle relaxation and circulation.

In shiatsu, the dog's torso, head, and limbs are massaged and stretched, with finger pressure applied to key points. There are no official studies of its success, but it is used widely to promote healing, relaxation, and muscle-tension release because it is based on modern knowledge of canine anatomy.

Other therapies

In addition to massage, many other therapies are helpful to dogs. Nutrition, herbalism, homeopathy, and Bach flower remedies are only a few. But not everything that works for people is suitable for dogs. Remember to ask for advice from canine therapists or vets who are sympathetic to complementary medicine.

Ben the scaredy-pooch

case history 4

Mary will always remember the moment when she first saw Ben at the animal rescue shelter. He was huddled at the back of the cage, a picture of misery, and shaking with fear. Immediately, Mary felt a rush of compassion for this frightened creature, and decided there and then that she was going to give him a home. She was confident that a loving family would transform Ben into a happy dog and an amiable companion.

Eventually, that did happen—but not without a few obstacles along the way. The rescue shelter didn't have much information about

Ben's previous experience—he'd been picked up from the street, and it looked like he'd been abandoned, or had simply strayed away from home. Mary noticed immediately that he was terrified of meeting new people and other pets. Taking him to the vet for the first time was a major operation—they both ended up as nervous wrecks. She wondered whether he had been physically abused in the past, his fear was so obvious.

Mary's neighbor Tom owned a friendly little mutt called Jodie, but when he tried to introduce her to Ben, he cringed, and shook with fear. Mary was very apologetic, but fortunately her neighbor was completely unfazed. "Why not try massage?" he said, "it's supposed to calm their nerves." Mary was so worried about Ben, she thought it was worth a try—and found a basic book at her local library.

After a few attempts, Mary soon found out the strokes Ben liked best. She also noticed that he was not only calmer, but began actually "asking" for massage. Then Mary's daughter learned how to massage Ben. Tom called over during one of these sessions, and Ben was so relaxed and happy, he even let Tom join in! "Jodie's going to get jealous—I'll have to wise up on this myself," laughed Tom. It wasn't too long before the two doggy neighbors became best friends, and enjoyed their walks and games together in the park. As for Ben's fear? In a while, he got much more confident, and was never called a scaredy-pooch again.

index

Published by MQ Publications Limited
12 The Ivories, 6–8 Northampton Street
London N1 2HY
Tel: +44 (0) 20 7359 2244
Fax:+44 (0) 20 7359 1616
email: mail@mqpublications.com
website: www.mqpublications.com

Copyright © MQ Publications Limited 2004
Text Copyright © 2004 Wendy Kavanagh
Illustrations Copyright © 2004 Bo Lundberg

Editor: Yvonne Deutch
Design: Lindsey Johns

ISBN: 1-84072-833-7

10 9 8 7 6 5 4 3 2 1

Printed and bound in China

This book contains the
opinions and ideas of the
author. It is intended to
provide helpful and informative
material on the subjects
addressed in this book and is
sold with the understanding
that the author and publisher
are not engaged in rendering
medical, health, or any other
kind of personal professional
services in this book. The
reader should consult his or
her medical, health, or
competent professional before
adopting any of the
suggestions in this book or
drawing references from it.
The author and publisher
disclaim all responsibility for
any liability, loss, or risk,
personal or otherwise, which
is incurred as a consequence,
directly or indirectly, of the use
and application of any of the
contents of this book.